Exercise

Top 20 Exercise Tips to Get in Shape

By

Bring on Fitness

About Bring On Fitness

Our passion for fitness gave life to **Bring On Fitness**. We started with the goal of helping as many people as we can. To educate, motivate and to help change peoples lives for the better. Bring On Fitness is not only for the fitness enthusiasts, but also for the beginner. We strongly believe nothing is more important than learning the basics and creating a strong foundation in both nutrition - through meal planning, and in exercise - by following a specific plan. This is just as important for the beginner, as it is for the experienced athlete.

We set high standards for ourselves, the information we share, and the products we carry. Our goal is to provide you with exceptional products that suit your needs and the knowledge and motivation to help you work towards and achieve your health and fitness goals.

Check us out at www.bringonfitness.com

"Our Mission is to have a positive impact in changing peoples lives. We will deliver the best possible fitness and nutrition solutions that will empower people to achieve their health and fitness goals."

Table of Contents

Introduction

Fitness is a key part of a healthy lifestyle, and this book will show you how to make the most of your time and environment when working out. These are tips to begin your journey, and we show you how to pump it up a notch along the way! This book is the first step to a new, healthier you!

Chapter 1: Preparation for the Beginner

Stop making excuses, and just begin!

We will address the most common excuses we all use to justify not beginning to get fit for real!

Tip #1: You can afford to go to the Gym

There are so many different types of gym memberships available that cost really shouldn't factor into the equation. For as little as $10 a month, you should be able to find a deal that suits your budget. Shop around and find a deal that you can afford, or even take up a 'free month" deal. There is bound to be one near you.

Alternatively, see if any of your friends are members of local gyms, and see if they can get you a guest pass so you can check out the facilities. If you are serious about increasing your fitness, you will be able to find a way. You don't need spend on a high monthly fee for a gym with a fancy pool area or a sauna if cost really is an issue.

You also really need to decide if it is the cost that is putting you off or the actual physicality of going to the gym. Sometimes the thought of exercising in front of others can be daunting. If that is the case, then think about investing in a few key pieces of equipment that will enable you to work out at home.

Tip #2: Take that first step

If you are too embarrassed to begin working out, then start with a walk! This is the first step for many people who have serious issues with their weight or fitness. Join a friend for a walk, and you may amaze yourself at the distance you cover.

Video workouts are a great way to exercise in the comfort of your own home, and there are plenty of different types that can be matched to your level of fitness. Choose a program that can advance with you and can be altered to match your ability and fitness levels.

Tip #3: Find a friend

Exercising can be a lonely experience and can require a huge supply of internal motivation, so hooking up with a fitness partner or even a group of people can be just the push you need to help you work out. Chatting and sharing your experiences can make the time fly by, and it is easier to give up if you are flying solo!

What if you don't have a friend who is into fitness? Well, instead of seeing this as a problem, you can always view it as an opportunity to make new friends. Try the bulletin board at work first, and see if any of your colleagues wish to join your new venture. If this is unsuccessful, then branch out and use social media to get your new partner in fitness!

There are apps out there that work like Tinder but pair you up with like-minded fitness partners. You may want someone who plays squash or tennis, as well as working out. You can use these apps to improve your sports and social life.

Tip #4: Commit for a set amount of time

When you commit yourself to a project, it is normal to have a time schedule in place. Working out is no different. Make sure you choose the length of time carefully, and do not pick an unrealistic target. There are many varied workout schedules available, and if you study them closely, the majority tend to advise you to commit for a minimum three months.

This is a lengthy time for many, and it may be advisable to choose a shorter time when you are beginning your new regime. A month is plenty of time to see if you can actually commit and is also the most common length of time for special offers at the gym. Mark the day you begin on a calendar or diary, or even in your media device, and then mark the calendar a month later. You may not be a gym buff after four weeks, but you will have a good idea of the level of fitness you wish to achieve.

Tip #5: Building your workout routine

There are many different aspects to consider when perfecting your workout routine. And it can be an intensely personal experience, but by considering different factors, you can tailor the routine that works best for you.

What are you doing at the moment? Consider what exercises you are doing regularly, and ask yourself if they are working for you. Do they challenge you? Are they helping you to improve your fitness? If they are tried and tested and you are comfortable with these exercises, then you must keep them.

Starting fresh

Begin by choosing the options that suit you best. These are not necessarily gym based and can include walking, dancing, swimming, cycling, and even gardening. So how long should you do it? It is recommended by the American Health Authority that we should be doing around 30 minutes a day of moderate exercise daily. This will help you get started, and you should see the benefits of regular movement quite quickly.

Ready to move on?

If you have any issues at all with your fitness and are unsure of how to begin your routine, you should check in with your doctor. Getting medical clearance is a must for anybody with health issues, but even if you are not in that category, you should at least monitor your heart rate when exercising.

Set your goals: Make sure your goals are clear and concise. There is no point in setting expectations that are unrealistic, as you will only disappoint yourself and run the risk of failure.

Start slow

Beginners often make the mistake of attempting workout movements that are beyond them. At best, they will be tired and sore while at worst; they run the risk of serious injury that will finish their training program before it even starts!

Aerobic or cardiovascular: These are great exercises for newbies and, simply put, are meant to speed up your breathing and heart rate. The exercises we mentioned earlier are great for these results. Walking, running, etc., will all help you to get into the routine of working out.

Tip #6: Set a schedule

So, now you have the beginnings of a workout routine in place, you are good to go, right? Wrong! You need to set your schedule and keep to it. If you do not have fixed times planned for your workouts, you easily run the risk of putting them off. Set your exercise routines to coincide with your regular free times, and you will more likely to stick to them. Plan your routine in advance, and ensure you factor in travel time and time to wash up or shower.

By considering your schedule and fitting your workouts to coincide with it, chances are you will stick to it and achieve success!

Make sure you allow for a warm up period before your session and a cool down period afterward. This may seem like a time-wasting exercise, but it is important to consider pre- and post-exercise activities as they lessen the chance of injury and can increase recovery times.

Chapter 2: Setting the Stage

Tip #7: Get the correct amount of sleep

It is often an overlooked fact that sleep plays a major part in a successful exercise routine, and it is essential that you achieve between seven and nine hours of quality sleep nightly. In order to achieve this rate of sleep, there are a few tricks we can use to help improve our sleep patterns.

Evaluate your room

The correct environment can aid in a good night's sleep, but it is a common mistake to consider simply the décor of your bedroom. Yes, it is important to use soothing colors and décor that contribute to your sleep quality, but you also need to consider the temperature of your room.

You should not be sleeping in a warm room; a cool bedroom will provide the best conditions, and you should strive to keep your bedroom between 60 and 65 degrees. If you need to use air conditioning or fans to do this, choose the quietest ones you can find.

The perfect bedroom should also be free of all light and, if necessary, you should wear eye shades or invest in blackout curtains.

Your bed

You need a comfortable and supportive mattress backed up by quality pillows. There are some effective anti-allergen pillows available if you have allergy issues, and these can be reasonably priced and available from all good outlets. Remember that your mattress has a shelf life and should be changed around every 10 years.

Remove the noise

Your sleep can be affected by distractions, such as electronic devices, and your sleeping area should be kept free of any device that is likely to make "white noise" during the night. Leave your smart devices outside the bedroom r turn airplane mode on.

Tip #8: Invest in a personal trainer

There are some of us who will need an extra push to achieve our fitness goals, and one answer can be to hire a personal trainer. This can be a great way to kick start the new super fit you, but first, you must consider the following criteria before choosing the right trainer for you:

Credentials

No matter what else you consider, there must be some certification to your trainer's skills. Make sure he or she has a recognized certificate from a credited organization.

Experience

This is a slightly trickier area as we would all prefer a trainer with experience and are reticent about using a newly qualified trainer. However, everyone must start somewhere, and enthusiasm may outweigh experience with a new trainer. You may also be able to strike a better deal with a less experienced person. You need to weigh the options carefully.

Specialty

Match your trainer with your personal needs. There is no point employing a trainer who is a running specialist if you are planning to concentrate on weight training.

Cost

It is all well and good to say you can't put a price on your fitness, but as this is going to be a relationship that can develop into a long-term situation, then cost has to be considered.

Personality

You need to get the trainer to suit you, and if you need a drill sergeant type of trainer, then make sure you get someone who will be pushing you to the very limit. Most of us, however, would prefer to have a positive relationship with our trainer. Positive reinforcement or military style – choose the personality that suits your needs.

Availability

In order to remove stressful situations, choose a trainer who is willing to fit in with your schedule. If you need to know exactly when your sessions will occur and prefer them to be rigidly maintained, then make sure you choose a trainer who can fit you in and will not cancel appointments. If you have a hectic schedule and need to be able to change your appointments weekly, make sure your potential trainer understands and is willing to juggle their time to fit your schedule. This can often be a crucial factor in the choice you are making.

Recommendations

Do not be lax when it comes to checking out their referrals. Unless they are newly certified, it should be a simple task to follow up on their present or former clients. If they seem unwilling to provide any sort of referral, then may be it is just best to walk away.

Tip #9: Give yourself a break

It is so tempting to begin your new exercise regime full steam ahead, but don't forget that your body needs a break! Make sure you take at least one full day a week without strenuous exercise, and listen to your body. Rest days are just as important as workout days, so avoid treating them as "slacking off," and allow yourself to recuperate properly. It is advised that if your body is not used to regular exercise, you should employ two out of three methods. Following two days of exercise, you should take a rest day.

You can still complete a mild form of exercise on a rest day, but it should be a fun activity. Try walking or playing golf to keep your body active. A well-earned rest day will enable you to jump right back into the program with a fresh sense of energy.

Tip #10: Start Small

Be cautious when you are assessing your fitness levels, and be honest with yourself on your limitations. If you embark on a program that you are not physically capable of, you run the risk of discouraging yourself and possibly quitting; as you may fail to meet your goals. It is better to underestimate your abilities and be amazed by what you are capable of rather than run the risk of disappointment.

It is a common mistake to set too many goals when beginning to exercise, so here are four important points that should be adhered to when considering your program.

1. **There is no such thing as "too easy":** You know what you are capable of, so aim just above it! Has it been years since you have exercised? If so, set yourself a goal of 10 minutes of brisk walking a day. You can do that, right? After two weeks, up it to 20 minutes. The goal is to build your habits and increase it when you are comfortable doing so.

2. **Name it:** Write down what you are going to do and when, and then leave that note where you can see it. For instance, instead of writing "exercise for 20 minutes," make sure you specify what you are doing; 'walk for 20 minutes, Monday from 3:00 to 3:20."

3. **Trigger points**: This is a great tip that can make your body recognize when it is time to exercise. Consider what triggers you already have. Do you have a shower and then immediately brush your teeth? That is a trigger, so doing the same activity directly before every exercise session can prepare your body for the workout to come. Do you have a coffee right before you work out? Great, that's your personal trigger, so use it!

4. **Numbers**: It is important to quantify your activities as it gives perspective, so instead of planning exercise times, try placing a numerical quantity to your goals. For example: Do three sets of 10 push-ups daily. Run for a mile. Walk for three miles. Using specific numbers

allow you to view your goals in a different manner and choose how you achieve them.

Chapter 3: Moving Forward

You are now at the point in which you are in full swing with your new regime and are committed to your program. So you are feeling good and looking well, right? Here are a few problems that you may be experiencing and how to overcome them.

Tip #11: Patience

How many times have you heard a "fitness guru" promising you that you will have the perfect beach body by summer, or that you can become pumped in a month? These are blatant untruths that are merely touted in order to promote a product or service. The reality is that deciding to get fit is a long-term commitment and, even when you feel like you have put the work in but are not seeing the results, you must still keep at it!

Working out is a process that involves many highs and lows, and the trick is to power through the lows and celebrate the highs. Your body needs constant coaxing, and you need the patience to keep going even when life drops obstacles in your way.

Do not fall into the trap of comparing your progress with people who have been working out for years. There is a good reason they look the way they do, and the reason is consistency! If you aspire to reach a similar physique, be realistic about the time required. So stay focused and keep pushing forward!

Tip #12 New Rewards

So you have reached a number of goals, and you are feeling quite pleased with yourself. Feel like you are due for a treat or reward of some sort? Well obviously, you should break out the fast food, or maybe a huge ice cream cake to treat yourself! But surely, that will leave you feeling guilty and bloated, so how about taking a new look at a reward for yourself?

Treat yourself to some new gym gear. There are some really stylish brands you can choose from when you are looking at workout clothing. Spend some cash on a new outfit or gym shoes, and avoid the guilt trip that some rewards can cause. Maybe you have always wanted to start a home gym – look into some equipment for your home.

Buy a set of dumb bells and use them at home. Whatever you decide, the main thing is to change your attitude toward rewards. They do not have to be unhealthy or bad for you. You are changing your attitude, as well as your body, so think healthy and stay healthy.

Tip #13: Track your body

It is important to track your progress correctly, and quite often, this involves numerous readings and measurements. The scales do not tell the whole story, and quite often, people can get disillusioned when their weight is not falling off as quickly as they expect. The truth is that if you are working out properly and tracking your changes correctly, you will soon realize that you are making significant progress in other healthier areas.

Tracking your body is important but should not be done on a daily basis. Bodies fluctuate and can give inaccurate information if the timing is wrong, so here are a few alternative methods to track your progress that you can use, along with your weight scales!

- **The camera never lies:** In the beginning taking pictures of your body can be difficult, but you should stand in front of a full-length mirror and take a picture. Oh, and you should be in your underwear! Tough for some, but you must do it to get a true picture of what you are trying to achieve. Remember to take a side profile and then keep the photos ready for comparison.
- **Measure:** Use a tape measure to track your progress but don't just concentrate on your waist or hips. Use the tape to measure the circumference of these areas, and you will be amazed at the changes.

  - Neck – between the head and the shoulders
  - Shoulder – place both arms down by your side, and measure the widest point from one shoulder to the other
  - Bicep – the top of your arm
  - Thigh – left or right, but be consistent

  Always measure before you work out; make sure you are taking the readings from the same spot every time. Use freckles or moles whenever possible to know exactly where to measure.

- **Body fat:** There are two approaches to consider when measuring body fat, but they differ in accuracy, so the choice is yours. You can purchase a body fat caliper for a small amount of cash, and measure your own progress. It is important to realize that the readings are less than accurate, and the best way to use them is to take multiple readings and gather an average. When tracked this way, the best you can hope for is to indicate a trend, and make sure you are heading in the right direction.

If body fat measurement is important to you, then you may consider paying for it to be measured by a professional. This will cost around fifty dollars a session, but if you get it measured every two months, this can be a wise investment.

Tip #14: Compound Exercises

As you become more comfortable in your training, it will benefit you to begin compound exercises instead of focusing on isolation exercises. So, what is the difference?

Simply put, isolation exercises involve one muscle group at a time, and compound exercises involve multiple joints and multiple muscle groups.

Examples of compound exercises are:

- **Bench press**: All forms of bench press are compound exercises and you can try the barbell and flat forms to improve your chest, shoulder, and triceps.
- **Pull up**: This is a simple move that involves the biceps and forearms and can be done almost anywhere.
- **Rowing**: Take advantage of the rowing machine and you will be exercising your back, biceps, and forearms.
- **Squat**: The simple squat and its variations – front, back, and split – will activate over 200 muscles at a time, but when properly executed, it improves the calves, glutes, hamstring, and thigh muscles.

The bottom line is that when executed correctly, you can use compound exercises to improve your results as exercise multiple muscles at the same time.

Tip #15: Accept discomfort

Physical activity will always produce discomfort, and it is crucial to know the difference between discomfort and pain. Knowing when to stop is key to working out healthily. When we exercise, our muscles produce lactic acid, and this is what causes the "burn" that we all know accompanies exercise. While it is normal to feel discomfort and aches when exercising, if the pain develops into a stabbing or sharp pain, this could be a sign to stop.

Chest pains are also an indication to stop your workout and should never be ignored. Listen to your body, and learn the difference between "good pain" and signs that you are overdoing it. If it feels like you are doing too much, then ease off. Always give your body time to rest when it is telling you it needs it. After a couple of days, you should feel ready to resume.

Chapter 4: The Next Step

Now, we are ready to intensify our workout experience. These last few tips will set you on the path to a healthier, fitter future for the new you.

You may be finding that you are spending significant time in the gym, and you need to cut back on that time while maintaining the intensity of your exercises. This is the time to consider high-intensity interval training.

Tip #16: High-intensity Interval Workouts

These workouts are designed to get you in and out of the gym as quickly as possible; you are aiming to get your heart rate close to its maximum, and then rest briefly before doing it all over again. You can accomplish a higher level of exercise in a shorter time and increase your aerobic capacity at the same time.

Try these simple high-intensity interval workouts, and push yourself to the next level.

Sprint and walk

It really is as simple as it sounds. Start with a 20-second walk, followed by a 20-second sprint, and repeat up to 10 times. This should create the burn andyou're your heart rate up. The first few times you do it, you may feel like giving up half way through, but push on, and you will reap the rewards. This simple workout can be adjusted to suit any age or fitness level.

If needed it after the 20-second walk, sprint for 10-seconds; and gradually build up your sprint time.

Infinite pushups

Sounds like fun, right? Yeah, I know, but try it anyway. Do 10 pushups at a time and then rest, again repeat up to 10 times. Optimum rest time is around 30 seconds, but you can tailor this to fit your fitness level by resting more if needed. The same applies to the number of reps you do, 10 can be reduced and gradually build up.

Infinite squats

Follow the same program that you did with the pushups, and you will soon see the benefits. Do 10 squats and rest; then, repeat and rest up to 10 times. You get the picture, right?

Jog and sprint

This is like the first exercise, but you will replace the walk with a jog. This is a great way to increase your aerobic capacity.

There are many more combinations of exercise that are classified as high-intensity interval training, and as you improve your level of fitness, you can combine them to push your body even further. The key is to understand the concept of short burst exercises followed by rest periods.

Tip #17: Power up your run

The run can be a core part of your exercise regime, but how can you power it up to optimize the time you spend running? Try incorporating exercise drills when running, and you will add interest, as well as extra exercise.

Use squats and lunges to break up a run, and also try some full body moves, such as the push-ups or burpees.

If you are uneasy adding moves to your run, then consider the environment you are in. If you run solely on a track, maybe it's time to take up uphill running. Whatever you choose, make sure it is a forward step in your fitness plan.

Tip #18: Try something new

This is a great time to up your game, and take on another activity. You are feeling fitter and healthier so why not consider something that would have been beyond the pre-workout you? Rock climbing is a great activity to test your new fitness levels, especially arm and leg strength.

Take on challenges that you would have dismissed before – maybe a half marathon or a sponsored bike ride. Leave the unadventurous you behind, and take on the world!

Tip #19: Stretch at Work

Depending on your workplace, there is always a chance to exercise, no matter how sedentary your job is. If you are seated at a desk for long periods of time, then stretching is the least you can do.

Interlace your fingers, and stretch up to the ceiling, try combining with some vigorous shrugs, and you will feel your upper arm area growing stronger.

Hugging your knee and bringing it up to chest level will help you exercise your leg muscles. Hold this position for 10 seconds, and then repeat with your other leg.

Extend your arm, and reach out as far as you can in the opposite direction. Hold for a few seconds and then make sure you do it with the other arm.

Tip #20: Don't skimp on carbs

When you are pushing your body toward fitness, it is important that you are fueling it correctly. This requires you to stock up on carbohydrates, but you need to know the "good" carbs from the "bad" carbs.

Good Carbs

Known simply as whole carbs, these are the fibers found naturally in food and should be used to fuel your workouts. Examples include fruit and vegetables; potatoes and grains also contain healthy carbs.

Bad Carbs

These are also referred to as refined carbs and include sugary drinks and bread. The general rule is that white is bad! White bread, rice, or pasta should all be avoided and replaced with wholegrain alternatives. Refined carbs are responsible for elevated blood sugar levels that can lead to hunger cravings and can create a blood sugar roller coaster.

These carbs are also known as empty carbs and provide no nutrition whatsoever. The bottom line is that you should choose your carbs carefully, and avoid refined versions. Choose the unprocessed carbs for optimum health benefits.

Conclusion

Now, you have a chance to change your life and embark on a healthy new lifestyle. Grab it with both hands, and make those changes. Good luck with your new life and your positive new attitude toward exercise.

Thank you, and remember to share how well these exercise tips work for you. You can do that here...

Thank you,

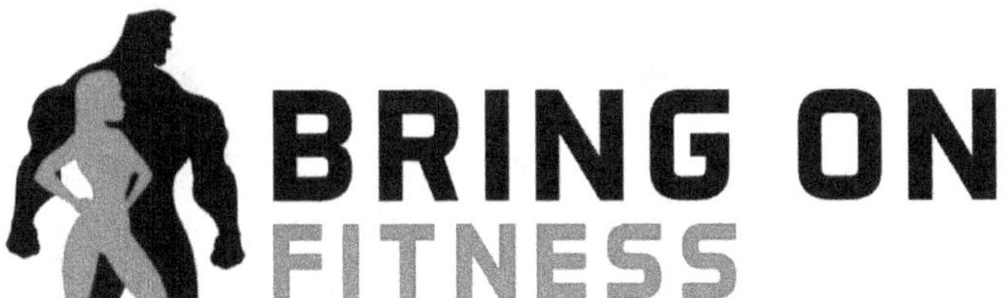

Acknowledgments

http://effectivehiitworkouts.com

http://nerdfitness.com

https://www.healthline.com